Easy Gout Cookbook

30 Easy Recipes That Could Aid in A Gout Cure

An all-Natural and Delicious Gout Remedy

BY

Gordon Rock

Copyright 2016 Gordon Rock

License Notes

No part of this Book can be reproduced in any form or by any means including print, electronic, scanning or photocopying unless prior permission is granted by the author.

All ideas, suggestions and guidelines mentioned here are written for informative purposes. While the author has taken every possible step to ensure accuracy, all readers are advised to follow information at their own risk. The author cannot be held responsible for personal and/or commercial damages in case of misinterpreting and misunderstanding any part of this Book

About the author

Gordon Rock is the author for hundreds of cookbooks on delicious meals that the 'average Joe' can attempt at home. Including, but definitely not limited to, the Amazon Prime bestseller "Smoking Meat: The Essential Guide to Real Barbecue".

Rock is also known for other well-known titles such as "Making Fresh Pasta", "Hot Sauce", "The Paleo Chocolate Lovers" and "Vegan Tacos", just to name a few.

Rock has been nominated for various awards and has recently been offered a 'Question & Answers' column in Food and Wine Magazine that will give him a greater medium to respond to all the queries readers may have after attempting his recipes. He has also been honored by the

Institution of Culinary Excellence for his outstanding recipes.

Gordon Rock grew up in the outskirts of Los Angeles in California, where he graduated from the Culinary Institute of America with honors. He still resides there along with his wife and three kids. He operates a non - profit organization for aspiring cooks who are unable to finance their culinary education and spends practically all his spare time either in the kitchen or around his desk writing.

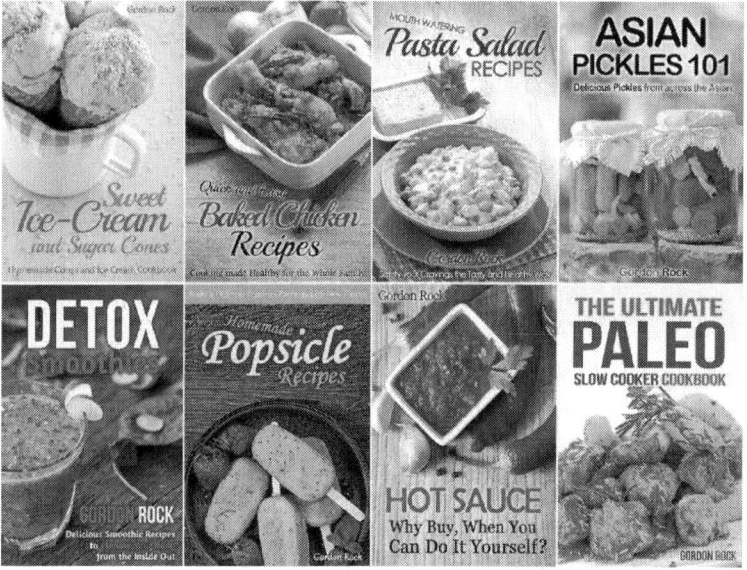

For a complete list of my published books, please, visit my Author's Page...

http://amazon.com/author/gordonrock

You can also check out my blog at: http://grodon-rock.blogspot.com

Or my Facebook Page at:
https://www.facebook.com/ChefGordonRock

Table of Contents

Introduction 8
What is Gout and what causes it? 10
Appetizer Recipes 12
    Curried Carrot, Sweet Potato, and Ginger Soup 13
    Waldarf Salad 15
    Cucumber Yogurt Salad 17
    Garlic Red Potato Salad 18
    Roasted Potatoes with Onion & Rosemary 19
    Green Bean and Macaroni Salad 21
    Asian-Inspired Chicken Wings 23
    Moo Shu Chicken Wraps 25
Main Course Recipes 27
    Gout Friendly Oven Baked Arancini Balls 28
    Chicken and Cornmeal Dumplings 30
    Apricot Tequila Glazed Drumsticks 32
    Caribbean Dump Chicken 34
    Chicken Stuffing Casserole 36
    Skillet Chicken Bulgogi 37
    Split Pea Soup 38
    Thai Peanut Chicken 39
    Curry Chicken Stew 41
    Thai Chicken Soup 43
    Thai Vegetable Curry 45

- Lentil Slow Cooker Chowder 47
- Fruit Water & Drinks Recipes 49
  - Raspberry Cacao Blast..50
  - Watermelon Minty Water 51
  - Zesty Mango Water...52
  - Raspberry Orange Water..53
  - Lemon Berry Mixed Water 54
  - Tropical Water 55
  - Refreshing Peach Water..56
  - Jamaican Carrot Juice Recipe 57
  - Jamaican Sour Sop Juice...58
  - Jamaican Sorrel Recipe..59
- Author's Afterthoughts..61

Introduction

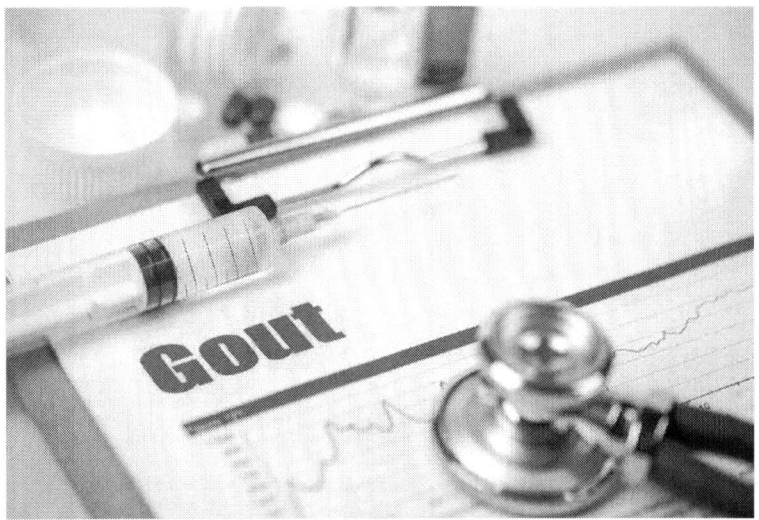

Congratulations on taking your first step to recovery! You are about to embark on a fun and delicious journey that will teach you how to better understand Gout, as well as, how to use small changes in your daily diet to combat the disease. While doing so you will be introduced to some new interesting ingredients that will help you realise that there are healthy ways to enjoy similar delicious meals you are used to.

These are recipes I discovered myself after being diagnosed with arthritis a little under a month ago and was forced to make a drastic lifestyle change in order to lower my uric acid levels. Being a foodie, myself this was definitely a challenge at first but it gave me a chance to explore new foods, and there is nothing more exciting than discovering something new and delicious. These are the same recipes, explanations and tips that I will be sharing with you so that you too can live in the know and get rid of those horrible pain spasms once and for all. So let's jump right in by helping you understand what exactly Gout is and what causes it.

What is Gout and what causes it?

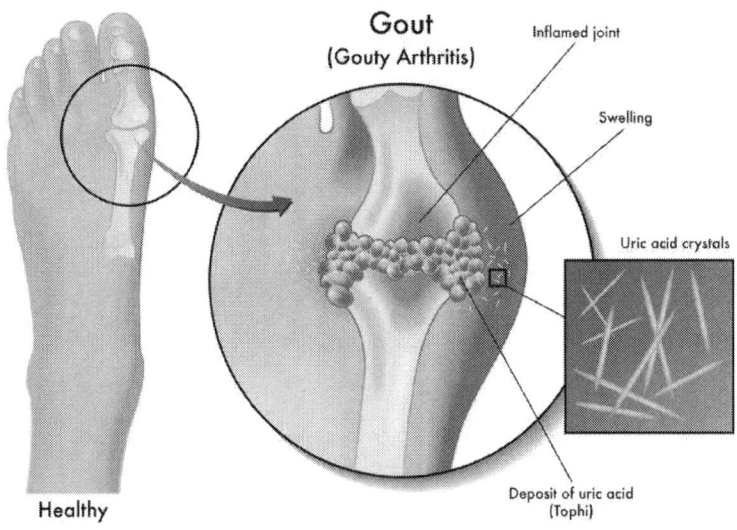

Gout, informally referred to the 'disease of the rich' is a branch of arthritis that develops as a result of there being too much uric acid in the body's blood stream. The body generally creates and uses uric acid from a substance called purines. Purines are found in most food and drinks that we intake and produced by the chemical breakdown of digestion. From here, the body uses what it needs and excretes the excess through urine. There are, however, a few cases in which the body for whatever reason is unable to excrete this excess so the body begins storing unnecessary uric acid. This unnecessary build up, over time, leads to joint swelling, inflammation of the joints and in turn extreme pain. All together these symptoms lead to the arthritis known as Gout.

The good news is there are certain lifestyle and dietary changes that can be made in order to control, and maybe even cure Gout. You will still need to take your medication as directed by your doctor, but avoiding certain foods such as red meat, sugary drinks, alcohol, acidic fruits/vegetables, certain gluten based products, and shellfish will vastly aid in you controlling the disease, and minimizing the pain you feel. By now you must be wondering after eliminating all that what will you be allowed to eat. Let's explore some recipes of dishes that will fit perfectly in your new lifestyle and still fulfilling your need for delicious food.

Appetizer Recipes

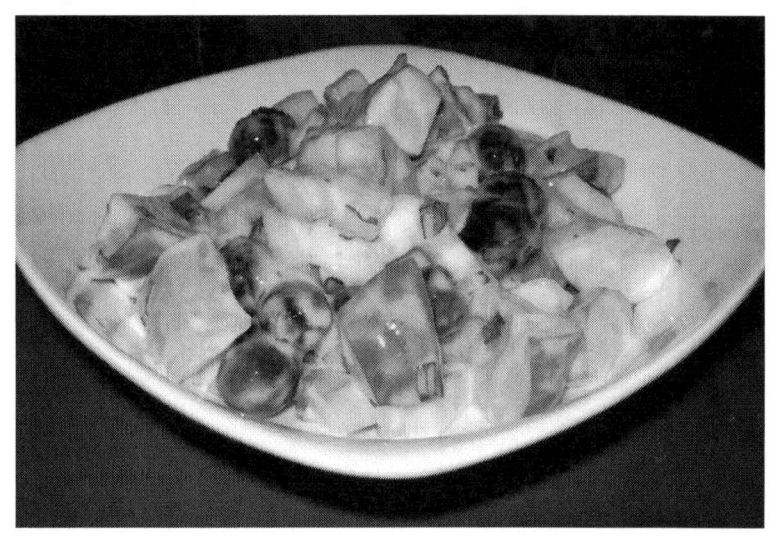

Curried Carrot, Sweet Potato, and Ginger Soup

Cholesterol isn't an issue when enjoying this delicious creamy soup, as it is filled with Beta-Carotene, and Vitamin A which together helps to promote healthy vision.

Yields: 5 Servings (1¼ cup per Serving)

Time Needed: 30 – 35min.

Ingredients:

- Extra Virgin Olive Oil (2 tsp.)
- Shallots (½ cup, chopped)
- Sweet Potato (3 cups, peeled, cubed)
- Carrots (1½ cup, peeled, sliced)
- Ginger (1 tbsp., grated)
- Curry Powder (2 tsp.)
- Chicken broth (3 cups, fat free)
- Salt (¼ tsp.)

Directions:

Place a saucepan with your oil on medium heat until it just begins to smoke. Add your shallots to the pot and sauté until it becomes tender (should take approximately 2 – 3 min). Add to the shallots all your prepped vegetables, and your curry then allow to cook for another 2 minutes. Pour in your broth and allow it to come to a boil. Once boiling, place the lid on the pot and reduce the heat to low. Allow this mixture to simmer until your vegetables are all tender. Once tender, add salt and pour your soup into a food processor. Pulse until creamy and smooth. Serve and Enjoy.

Tip: Consider topping with a teaspoon of vanilla Greek yogurt and sesame seeds.

Waldarf Salad

This delicious mix of fruits, nuts, and low – fat mayonnaise is the perfect snack for any time of the day.

Yields: 4 servings (1 cup of salad and 2 lettuce leaves per serving)

Time Needed: 5 min

Ingredients:

- Mayonnaise (2 tbsp., low-fat)
- Lemon Juice (1 tbsp.)
- Apples (2 Fuji, small, cubed)
- Grapes (1 cup, red, halves)
- Cranberries (1/3 cup, dried)
- Walnuts (1/4 cup, chopped)
- Celery (1/4 cup, sliced)
- Lettuce (8 leaves, Boston)

Directions:

Create a dressing in a medium bowl by whipping the lemon juice and mayonnaise until fully combined. Add your fruits, walnuts and celery to the dressing and mix until fully coated. Using 2 lettuce leaves per plate create beds on 4 plates and serve the salad on the lettuce beds. Enjoy.

Tip: If there is salad left over store in an airtight container in your refrigerator for up to 2 hours.

Cucumber Yogurt Salad

Snacks are the absolute hardest meal to plan within a gout diet as so many of the quick items are off your table of choices. Here is an easy and tasty snack that you can prepare for your entire family.

Yields: 4 – 6 Servings

Time Needed: 20 min

Ingredients:

- Greek Yogurt (2 cups, plain or vanilla)
- Cucumber (1 medium, peeled, thinly chopped)
- Mint (2 tablespoons, chopped thinly)
- Garlic Paste (1/4 tsp.)
- Salt (1/2 teaspoon)

Directions:

In a medium sized serving bowl thorough mix all the ingredients together until well incorporated. Place in the refrigerator to chill for at least 15 minutes. Serve and Enjoy!

Garlic Red Potato Salad

Here is a healthy version of a classic salad that will knock you out of your boots.

Yields: 2 – 4

Time Needed: 30 min

Ingredients:

- Red Potatoes (2 cups, diced, cooked)
- Garlic (8 cloves, crushed)
- Olive Oil (6 tablespoons)
- Greek Yogurt (1/2 cup, plain)
- Salt (1 teaspoon)
- Pepper (3/4 teaspoon)
- Green Onions (1 stalk, diced)
- Radishes (4, medium, sliced)
- Carrot (1 medium, diced)
- Sweet Pepper (1 medium, diced)

Directions:

In a large bowl, thoroughly combine all your ingredients until fully incorporated. Refrigerate and Serve. Enjoy!

Roasted Potatoes with Onion & Rosemary

This delicious meal is perfect for just a snack or even a delicious party starter.

Yields: 4 Servings

Time Needed: 35 min

Ingredients:

- Onion (1 small, chopped)
- Canola/Vegetable Oil (2 tbsp.)
- Rosemary (2 tbsp., chopped)
- Thyme (1 tsp., chopped)
- Salt (1/4 tsp.)
- Pepper (1/8 tsp.)
- Potatoes (1 ½ lbs., skin on, washed and cut into even chunks)

Directions:

Set your oven to preheat at 450 degrees F, and grease your baking sheet then set aside. In a large bowl create a rub by mixing together your rosemary, salt, pepper, onion, thyme and oil. Throw in your potatoes and toss until well coated. Line a ¬layer of potatoes onto your baking sheet ensuring that none overlaps. Bake until potatoes are tender and light brown in color.

Tip: Be sure to turn the potatoes occasionally. Cooking time could vary but generally takes 20 to 25 minutes to cook.

Green Bean and Macaroni Salad

A classic salad with a modern twist!

Yields: 4 -5 Servings

Time Needed: 15 minutes

Ingredients:

- Haricot Verts (1/4 cup, blanched and chopped in halves)
- Basil (1/2 cup, chopped)
- Macaroni (3 cups, cooked)
- Olive Oil (4 tbsp.)
- Garlic (2 cloves, crushed)
- Salt (3/4 tsp)
- Vinegar (2 tbsp.)
- Pepper (1/2 tsp.)

Directions:

In a small bowl, create a dressing by whipping together your vinegar, olive oil, garlic, salt and pepper. In another bowl add your remaining ingredients (macaroni, haricot verts, and basil) then pour the dressing over it. Toss until evenly coated. Serve and enjoy!

Tip: For an extra dash of protein or to transform into a main dish consider adding 1 cup of chickpeas to the salad before tossing.

Asian-Inspired Chicken Wings

Asian inspired wings that aren't sweet and sour or teriyaki but the fresh ingredients give it an Asian taste and feel that's to die for. If you can put these on the grill and barbecue them instead of baking they are even better.

Servings: 8

Preparation Time: 60 minutes

Carb: 8 g

Ingredients:

- Chicken Wings (3 lbs.)
- Extra Virgin Coconut Oil (2 tbsp.)
- Garlic (4 cloves, chopped)
- Ginger (1 tbsp., chopped)
- Anise Seed (1 tsp)
- Fennel Seed (1 tsp)
- Coconut Aminos (1/2 cup)
- Honey (2 tbsp.)
- Apple Cider Vinegar (2 tbsp.)
- Fish Sauce (1 tbsp.)
- Sesame Oil (2 tbsp.)

Directions:

Put wings into a large bowl, drain or pat to dry. In a small saucepan heat oil then add garlic, ginger, fennel seed and anise and cook for 3 minutes. Add honey, vinegar, aminos and fish sauce and cook for a minute. Remove from flame and add sesame oil. Pour mixture over wings and stir. Cool and refrigerate overnight, you may stir occasionally as it marinates. Remove wings from marinade and bake wings at 375 °until they are done. Remove from heat and enjoy. Add your favorite side dish or have as is.

Moo Shu Chicken Wraps

This Asian inspired wrap uses chicken moo shu instead of pork. The mixture is quick to put together and is rich in fiber.

Serves: 4

Preparation Time: 25 minutes

Ingredients:

- Chicken breasts (12 oz., halved)
- Olive oil (2 teaspoons)
- Onion (1, chopped)
- Black pepper (1/4 teaspoon)
- Corn Flour Tortillas (4 whole)
- Broccoli florets (2 cups)
- Ginger (1/2 teaspoon, ground)
- Hoisin sauce (3 tablespoons)

Directions:

1. Set oven to 350°F. Slice chicken into strips and put aside till needed. Put tortillas into foil, wrap and bake for 10 minutes until tortillas softened.

2. Heat half of oil in a skillet and add onion, pepper, broccoli and ginger to pot. Cook for 5 minutes then take vegetables from skillet and put aside.

3. Add leftover oil to skillet and heat then add chicken and cook for 5 minutes. Return vegetables to skillet along with hoisin sauce. Stir to combine and cook until thoroughly heated.

4. Spoon chicken mix into tortillas and roll. Slice in half and serve.

Main Course Recipes

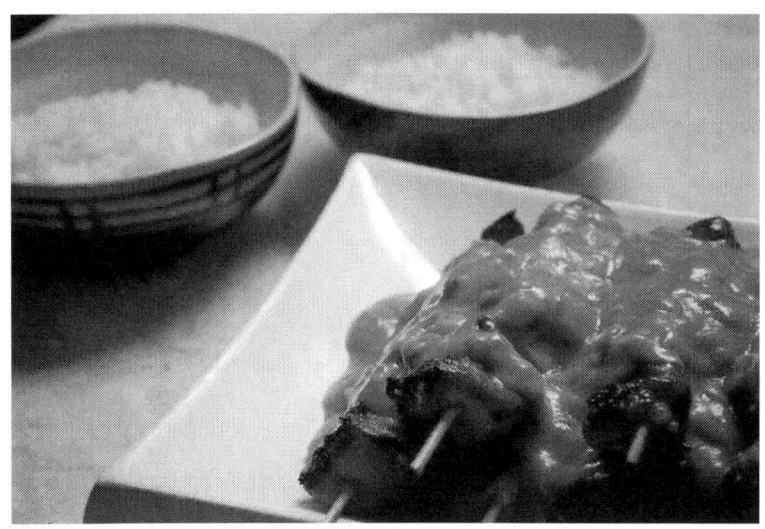

Gout Friendly Oven Baked Arancini Balls

Here is a gout friendly recipe to the Italian classic.

Yields: 12 Arancini balls

Time Needed: 30 minutes

Ingredients:

- Wineless Risotto (3 cups, chilled)
- Eggs (2, beaten)
- Gluten free Flour (1/4 cup)
- Cornmeal (1 ½ cups)

Directions:

Set your oven to preheat at 350 degrees F and grease a large baking sheet then line it with grease paper. Create a breading station by lining up your flour, eggs and cornmeal in 3 separate dishes. Proceed to roll scoops of risotto into balls about the size of a scoop of ice cream. Once formed, roll each ball into your flour until completely covered then dip the floured ball into your egg dish. Finally, remove the ball from the egg and roll it in cornmeal. Repeat this process until all your balls have been done. Next, line the balls up on your prepped baking sheet, gently spray with olive oil, and set to bake until the exterior is golden brown (should take approximately 15 - 20 minutes depending on your oven. Serve warm and enjoy.

Tip: Balls may be stuffed with mozzarella cheese when forming. May be served with lettuce cups, salad or jasmine rice.

Chicken and Cornmeal Dumplings

This one pot meal is full of protein and is bursting with flavor. These homemade dumplings are filling and pair deliciously with the chicken. Get that slow cooker out and try this wonderful meal.

Serves: 2

Preparation Time: 4-6 hours

Ingredients:

- Carrots (2, sliced thin)
- Corn kernels (1/3 cup)
- Garlic (2 cloves, diced)
- Black pepper (1/4 teaspoon)
- Chicken broth (1 cup, low salt)
- Oat Flour (1 tablespoon)
- Celery (1 stalk, sliced thin)
- Onion (1/2, sliced thin)
- Rosemary (1 teaspoon)
- Chicken thighs (2, skin removed)
- Milk (1/2 cup, fat free)

For dumplings:

- Oat Flour (1/4 cup)
- Baking powder (1/2 teaspoon)
- Egg white (1)
- Canola oil (1 tablespoon)
- Cornmeal (1/4 cup)
- Salt (1/4 tsp.)
- Milk (1 tablespoon, fat free)

Directions:

1. Prepare dumplings by combining flour, baking powder, salt and cornmeal in a bowl. Combine milk, oil and egg white in a separate bowl. Add wet mixture to dry mix and stir to combine until moist.

2. Add carrots, corn, garlic, black pepper, celery, onion and rosemary to slow cooker. Then put in chicken and broth.

3. Set on low and cook for 7-8 hours or on high for 3-4 hours.

4. Remove chicken from slow cooker and cool for 5 minutes then remove bones and chop chicken and return to cooker.

5. Combine flour and milk and add to slow cooker. Use spoon to drop dumplings into cooker. Cook for an additional 20-25 minutes.

Serve hot and enjoy!

Apricot Tequila Glazed Drumsticks

These glazed drumsticks are oh so yummy and are easy to whip up. The drumsticks are sweet and spicy and will become a favorite. These could replace traditional Buffalo wings and are crispy too.

Serves: 3

Preparation Time: 1 hour 10 minutes

Ingredients:

- Chicken drumsticks (6)
- Chile de arbol (2 tablespoons, crushed)
- Salt (1/4 tsp.)
- Apricot preserves (1 ½ cups)
- Sauza Tequila Blanco (1/3 cup)
- Black pepper (1/4 tsp.)

Directions:

1. Set oven to 350°F.

2. Combine chile de arbol, tequila and preserves in a saucepan and cook for 10 minutes over a low flame.

3. Use pepper and salt to season chicken and put into a baking dish.

4. Use sauce to coat chicken and pour leftover into dish.

5. Bake for 60 minutes until crisp and thoroughly cooked.

Caribbean Dump Chicken

Delicious chicken without the hassle with the wonderful aromas and flavors of the Caribbean islands.

Serves: 3 – 4

Time Needed: 4 - 6 hours

Ingredients:

- Brown sugar (1/4 cup)
- Orange juice (1/3 cup)
- Chicken parts (1 ½ lbs.)
- Pineapple chunks in juice (8 oz.)
- Nutmeg (1/2 teaspoon)
- Golden raisins (1/2 cup)

Directions:

1. Put all ingredients into a large Ziploc bag and combine.

2. Freeze overnight and remove the next day. Thaw completely.

3. Set slow cooker to high/ low

4. Add contents to bag and cook for 6-8 hours on low or 4-6 hours on high until thoroughly cooked.

Tip: Chicken may also be baked at 350°F for 30-60 minutes.

Chicken Stuffing Casserole

Enjoy the same homey taste with way less stress of it affecting your uric acid levels.

Serves: 3 – 4

Time Needed: 6 – 7 hours

Ingredients:

- Chicken breasts (4-6, deboned and skinned)
- Broccoli (10 oz., chopped)
- Chicken broth (1/2 cup)
- Gluten free Chicken stuffing (1 box)
- Cheesy broccoli soup (1 can)
- Butter

Directions:

1. Set slow cooker on low.

2. Use butter to grease slow cooker and then add chicken.

3. Combine all remaining ingredients and pour all over chicken.

4. Cover pot and cook for 6-7 hours.

Skillet Chicken Bulgogi

This is quite easy to make with delicious spices.

Serve: 3

Time Needed: 30 minutes

Ingredients:

- Chopped onion: ¼ cup
- Soy sauce: 5 tbsp.
- Minced garlic: 2 tbsp.
- Brown sugar: 2 ½ tbsp.
- Sesame oil: 2 tbsp.
- Sesame seeds: 1 tbsp.
- Cayenne: ½ tsp
- Salt and pepper
- Boneless chicken breasts, strips: 1 lb.

Directions:

1. Take a bowl and mix all ingredients except chicken.

2. Put chicken in mixture and coat well.

3. Take a skillet and transfer mixture with chicken into it. Cook on a medium heat for 20 minutes.

Split Pea Soup

Is there anything more comforting than a homemade soup? Only a split pea homemade soup.

Serves: 4

Time: 1 hour

Ingredients:

- 1 cup yellow split peas
- 4 cups vegetable broth
- ½ bay leaf
- ¼ teaspoon ground coriander seeds
- ½ tablespoon olive oil
- ½ teaspoon Salt
- ¼ teaspoon Pepper

Directions:

1. Rinse the peas under cold water and remove any black ones.

2. Place the rinsed peas into a rice cooker.

3. Add the remaining ingredients and give it a good stir.

4. Cover and cook for 60 minutes. Season to taste and serve while still hot.

Thai Peanut Chicken

Humble chicken combined with the zesty, crunchy, and fresh ingredients.

Serves: 8

Time: 4 hours 10 minutes

Ingredients:

- 4lb. skinless and boneless chicken breasts
- 2 tablespoons lime juice
- 1 cup chicken broth
- 4 tablespoon honey
- 1 cup peanut butter, preferably chunky
- 2 green bell peppers sliced
- 2 brown onions, diced
- 2 red bell peppers, sliced
- ½ cup fresh cilantro, chopped
- ½ cup soy sauce
- ½ cup crushed peanuts, for topping

Directions:

1. Place the sliced bell peppers and diced onion in the bottom of slow cooker.

2. Top with chicken breasts. You can either cut into larger chunks or place the whole breasts.

3. In a medium bowl, whisk the peanut butter, soy sauce, lime juice, honey, and chicken broth. Pour the prepared sauce over chicken.

4. Cook on high for 4 hours. During the last 15 minutes of cooking, shred the chicken with forks.

5. Continue cooking and once done serve with some hot rice or noodles.

6. Sprinkle with peanuts and chopped cilantro.

Curry Chicken Stew

Talking about the comfort food…this stew is perfect during the cold winter days and whenever you need something nourishing.

Serves: 4

Time: 4 hours 15 minutes

Ingredients:

- 5 chicken tights
- 5 chicken drumsticks
- 1 tablespoon Worcestershire sauce
- 14oz. can coconut milk
- ½ cup chicken stock
- 2 tablespoons fish sauce
- 2 tablespoons brown sugar
- 4 tablespoons red curry paste
- 1 tablespoon lemon juice
- 2 limes, juiced and zested
- 1 tablespoon olive oil
- ½ teaspoon Salt
- ¼ teaspoon Pepper

Directions:

1. Turn on the slow cooker.

2. Heat the oil in a skillet over medium-high heat. Season the chicken and cook in the oil until browned on all sides.

3. Remove and place in heated slow cooker.

4. Cook the curry paste in the same skillet for 1-2 minutes or until fragrant.

5. Add the Worcestershire sauce, brown sugar, and lemon juice. Cook until the sugar is melted.

6. Pour in the stock, coconut milk, fish sauce, lime juice, and zest.

7. Give it all a good stir and pour into the slow cooker. Cover and cook on high for 4 hours (low 8).

Tip: Serve with hot brown rice or gluten free noodles.

Thai Chicken Soup

Unlike the other staples of a Thai cuisine, this soup has milder aroma and is suitable for any occasion. The coconut milk gives it amazing aroma, while the peanut butter really smooths out the texture.

Serves: 4

Time: 4 hours 20 minutes

Ingredients:

- 0.5lb. roasted chicken carcass
- 14oz. can coconut milk
- 2 tablespoons smooth peanut butter
- ½ purple onion, sliced
- 2 tablespoons fish sauce
- 1 cup sliced shiitake
- 1 lime, juiced
- ¼ red bell pepper, sliced
- 2 tablespoons Thai curry paste
- 2 tablespoon brown sugar
- 1 tablespoon minced ginger
- Salt and pepper, to taste
- 3 cups water

Directions:

1. Place the chicken in a slow cooker and cover with water.

2. Season with salt and pepper and add the minced ginger.

3. Cover and cook on low for 4 hours.

4. Strain the stock through a fine sieve into a bowl.

5. Pull the meat off bones and return all to the slow cooker.

6. Add the remaining ingredients, except the lime juice.

7. Give it a good stir and cook for 15 minutes on high.

8. Turn off the heat and stir in the lime juice. Serve garnished with fresh chopped cilantro.

Thai Vegetable Curry

Who says that curry needs to be meat based? This recipe will allow you to enjoy a delicious a vegetable curry dish.

Serves: 4

Time: 8 hours 10 minutes

Ingredients:

- 2 cups cooked rice
- 14 oz. can diced tomatoes, with juices
- 1 teaspoon ground coriander seeds
- 2 tablespoons yellow curry paste
- 4 garlic cloves, minced
- 15 oz. chickpeas, rinsed
- 2 tablespoons quick cooking tapioca
- ½ lb. green beans, cut into ½-inch pieces
- 1 cup finely chopped brown onion
- 4 small carrots, chopped
- 2 medium potatoes, cut into ½-inch slices
- ½ teaspoon cayenne pepper
- 1 ½ cup vegetable stock
- 1 cup coconut milk
- Fresh ground salt and pepper
- 1/8 teaspoon cinnamon

Directions:

1. Combine all ingredients in a 4-quart slow cooker, except stock and tomatoes.

2. Blend ingredients well and pour in vegetable stock.

3. Cover and cook on low for 8 hours.

4. Stir in the tomatoes, with juices and cook additionally for 7 minutes.

Tip: May be served with cooked rice.

Lentil Slow Cooker Chowder

Lentils are a valuable source of proteins and vitamins and should be consumed whenever you can. With great recipes like this one, you will start to love the lentils, even if you are not already a big fan.

Serves: 4

Time: 5 hours 30 minutes

Ingredients:

- 1 cup red lentils
- 14oz. can coconut milk
- 1 cup water
- 1 ½ tablespoon yellow curry paste
- 3 garlic cloves, minced
- ¼ cup orange juice
- ½ cup diced tomatoes
- ½ cup diced potatoes
- 1 tablespoon dried parsley
- ¼ teaspoon fresh thyme
- 1 tablespoon minced ginger
- 2 teaspoons sugar
- 1 teaspoon hot sauce
- Salt and pepper- to taste

Directions:

1. Place lentils in the slow cooker.

2. Add the garlic, potatoes, ginger, sugar, hot sauce, and curry paste.

3. Pour the orange juice and water.

4. Cover and cook on high for 4-5 hours.

5. Add the remaining ingredients and cook for 20 minutes more.

6. Serve while still hot.

Fruit Water & Drinks Recipes

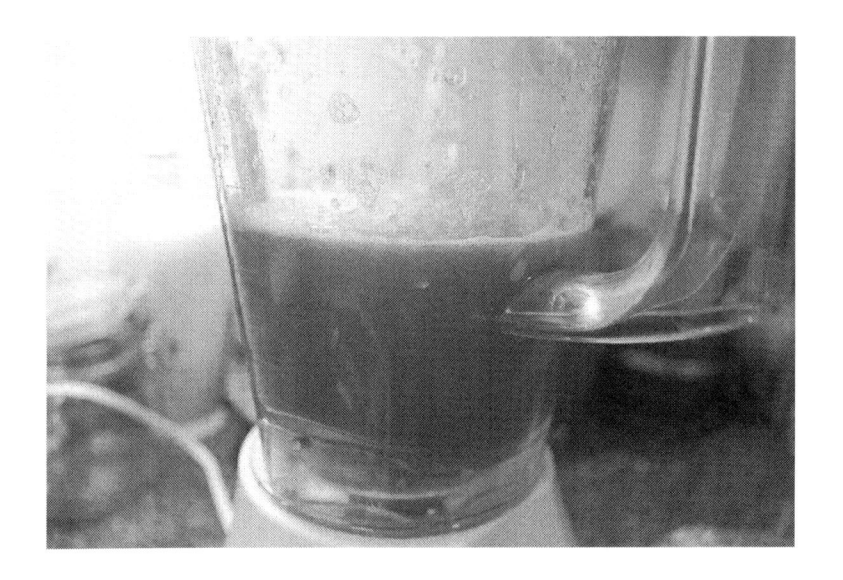

Raspberry Cacao Blast

Simple yet delicious summer smoothie.

Serves: 1

Time: 5 minutes

Ingredients:

- 1 cup raspberries
- 1 dash stevia powder
- 1 tablespoon raw cacao nibs
- 1 tablespoon Chia seeds
- 1 dash cinnamon
- Almond milk to max line

Directions:

Place raspberries, cacao nibs, Chia seeds and cinnamon in the blender. Add enough almond milk to reach the max line. Process for 30 seconds or until you get smooth mixture. Serve immediately in chilled tall glass.

Watermelon Minty Water

Refreshing, simple, sweet and delicious.

Makes: 64 fl. oz.

Time: 5 minutes + inactive time

Ingredients:

- 2 cups diced watermelon
- 4 mint leaves
- 8 cups water

Directions:

1. Remove any watermelon seeds.

2. Place all the ingredients into a pitcher.

3. Refrigerate for 2-24 hours.

4. Serve after.

Zesty Mango Water

The Mango-Ginger water that will refresh you up, while detoxifying the body.

Makes: 64 fl. oz.

Time: 5 minutes + inactive time

Ingredients:

- 1 cup diced mango
- 1-inch ginger, peeled and sliced
- 2 cups ice
- Water, to top off

Directions:

1. Peel and slice the ginger in 3-4-coin size slices.

2. Transfer the ginger into a pitcher along with mango.

3. Top with 2 cups ice and fill with water.

4. Refrigerate for 3 hours.

5. Serve after.

Raspberry Orange Water

Raspberries and oranges are everlasting combination and are great in any form, even infused water.

Makes: 48fl. oz.

Time: 5 minutes + inactive time

Ingredients:

- 2 mandarin oranges, cut into wedges
- ½ cup raspberries
- 6 cups water

Directions:

Place all the ingredients into a pitcher. Cover and refrigerate at least 2 hours or overnight. Serve after.

Lemon Berry Mixed Water

There is a good reason why this combination is commonly used in desserts: it is absolutely delicious as you will discover.

Makes: 24 fl. oz.

Time: 5 minutes + inactive time

Ingredients:

- 3 cups water
- 1 lemon, sliced
- ½ cup blueberries
- ½ cup raspberries

Method:

1. Combine all the ingredients into a pitcher.

2. Refrigerate for 2 hours or overnight.

3. Serve in the morning and drink through the day

Tropical Water

"Not only delicious, but also beneficial" is the sentence we can use to describe this infused water.

Makes: 64 fl. oz.

Time: 5 minutes + inactive time

Ingredients:

- ½ cup peeled and thinly sliced pineapple
- 1 orange, thinly sliced
- 2 cups ice
- Water, to top off

Directions:

1. In a large pitcher, combine the pineapple and orange.

2. Top with ice.

3. Pour in water to the top and cover.

4. Refrigerate for 1 hour before serving.

Refreshing Peach Water

When it is really hot outside and you need something that will cool you off, then prepare this amazing infused water.

Makes: 48 fl. oz.

Time: 5 minutes + inactive time

Ingredients:

- 10 frozen peach slices
- 1 sprig mint
- 1 cup ice
- 3 cups water

Directions:

Drop the peaches and mint into a large pitcher. Cover with ice and add water. Refrigerate for 4 hours before serving.

Tip: Drink throughout the day.

Jamaican Carrot Juice Recipe

A great accompaniment to a Sunday Dinner. This creamy juice is always a hit with diners of all ages.

Serves: 12

Time Needed: 20 minutes

Ingredients:

- Carrots (2 lbs)
- Water (5 cups)
- Milk (1 Cup, condensed)
- Nutmeg (1 tsp., grated)
- Vanilla (1 tsp.)

Directions:

Peel all your carrots and cut the peeled carrots into cubes. Pour you cut carrots into a blender with 1 cup of water and blend. Pass the blended mixture through your strainer to get the juice from it. Catch the juice into a container and discard the remaining pulp. Sweeten the juice with your milk and vanilla then mix well until fully combined. Add your nutmeg and lightly mix. Place in the freezer to chill for 1 – 2 hours. Serve chilled over ice.

Jamaican Sour Sop Juice

This is an easy drink to make and it's extremely delicious.

Serves: 12

Time Needed: 20 minutes

Ingredients:

- Sour Sop (1, ripe)
- Water (3 cups)
- Milk (1 Cup, condensed)
- Nutmeg (1 tsp., grated)
- Vanilla (1 tsp.)
- Crushed Ice (1 cup)
- Lime Juice (½ tsp.)

Directions:

Peel and cut up your sour sop. Place your soursop pieces (with seeds) into blender with 3 cups of water and blend on low speed for 2 seconds. Catch the juice into a container and discard the remaining seeds and pulp. Sweeten the juice with your milk and vanilla then mix well until fully combined. Add your nutmeg and lime juice then lightly mix. Place in the freezer to chill for 1 – 2 hours. Serve chilled over ice.

Jamaican Sorrel Recipe

This refreshing drink is often had at Christmas time with the family meal and can be had with or without rum.

Serves: 12

Time Needed: 24 hours & 20 minutes

Ingredients:

- Sorrel (3lbs)
- Ginger (1 inch, washed and crushed)
- Cloves (12)
- Pimento (4, green, dried grains)
- Cinnamon leaves (6)
- Boiling water (6 pt.)
- Granulated sugar (½ cup)
- Rice (1 tbsp.) optional

Directions:

1. Cut away the sepals of the sorrel from the seeds then wash well.

2. In a crock jar, add sepals, cloves, ginger, cinnamon leaves, rice and pimento.

NB: The rice here is optional as it's just used to increase the rate of fermentation. You may opt to omit the rice and allow the sorrel to stand longer than 24 hours.

3. Pour boiling water over this mixture, cover and let stand for 24 hours.

4. Strain the mixture and sweeten the juice with sugar.

6. Allow to chill for 1 – 2 hours.

7. Served chilled over ice.

Author's Afterthoughts

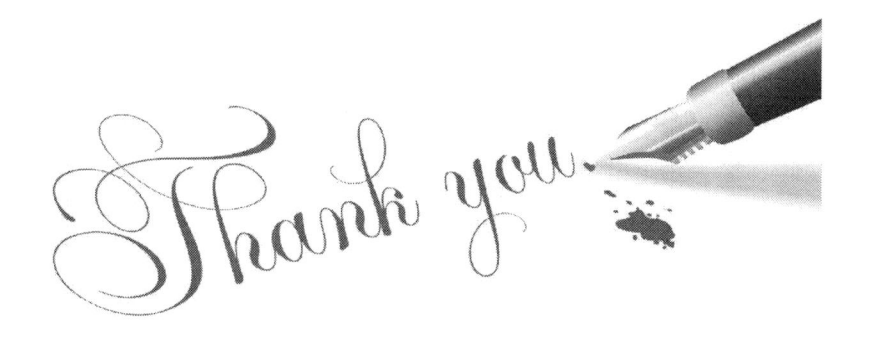

Thanks ever so much to each of my cherished readers for investing the time to read this book!

I know you could have picked from many other books but you chose this one. So a big thanks for downloading this book and reading all the way to the end.

If you enjoyed this book or received value from it, I'd like to ask you for a favor. Please take a few minutes to post an honest and heartfelt review on Amazon.com. Your support does make a difference and helps to benefit other people.

Thanks for your Reviews!

Gordon Rock
bunsomsaetow@gmail.com

Made in the USA
Middletown, DE
20 July 2018